TYPE 2 DIABETES COOKBOOK FOR KIDS

Fun & Flavorful Recipes to Empower Kids on Their Diabetes Journey

T. John

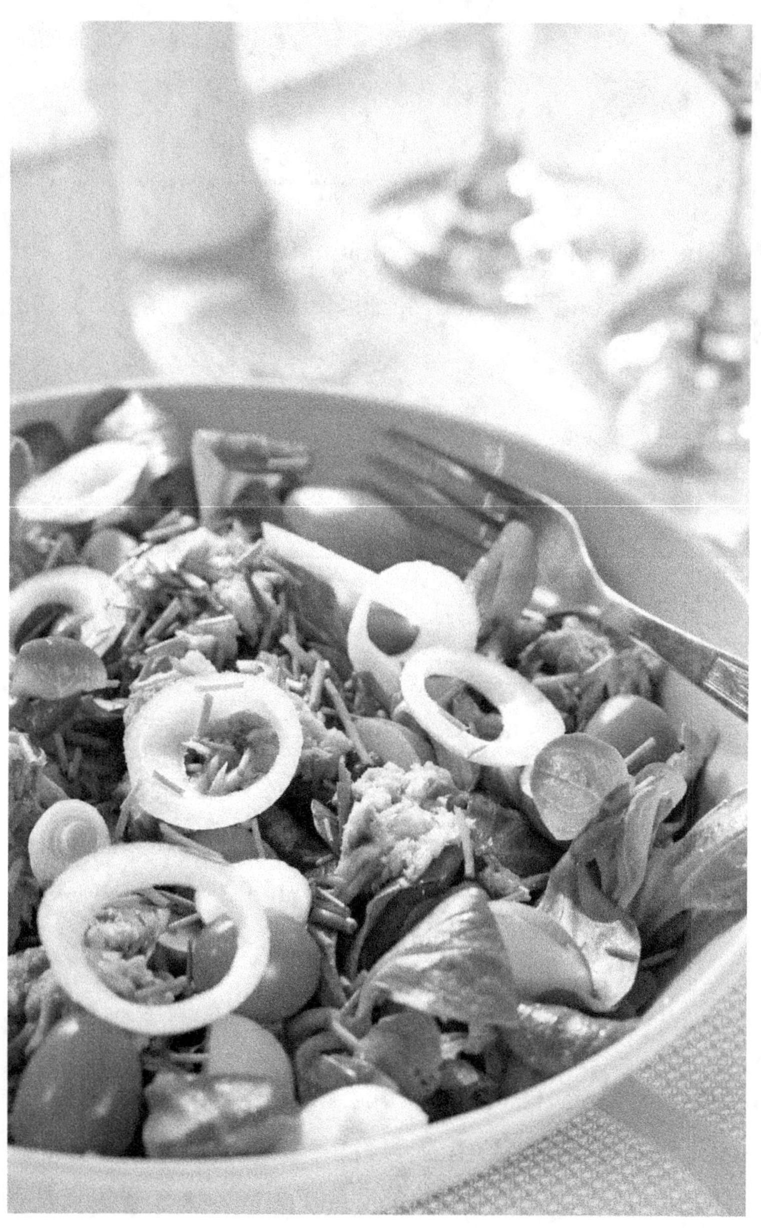

TABLE OF CONTENTS

Chapter 3: Lunch Recipes 45

Chapter 4: Dinner Recipes 69

Chapter 5: Snacks and Appetizers 96

Chapter 6: Desserts 112

INTRODUCTION

I magine your child, a ball of boundless energy, suddenly seeming sluggish. Maybe they're extra thirsty or have to use the restroom more often. These could be signs of type 2 diabetes, a condition where the body struggles to use sugar (glucose) for energy.

Here's a breakdown to help you understand what's happening:

- **The Body's Fuel Gauge:** Food is broken down into glucose, the body's fuel. Normally, the pancreas produces insulin, a key that unlocks cells, allowing glucose to enter and be used for energy.
- **The Glitch**: In type 2 diabetes, the pancreas either doesn't make enough insulin, or the cells become resistant, making it hard for glucose to enter. This leads to high blood sugar levels.

Why is this happening in kids?

Unlike type 1 diabetes, which is often genetic and affects insulin production, type 2 diabetes is linked to lifestyle factors. The rise in childhood obesity is a significant risk factor.

The Importance of Healthy Eating:

Just like filling your car with the right fuel, healthy eating is crucial for managing type 2 diabetes in children. Here's how:

- **Think Colorful Plate:** Fill half the plate with non-starchy vegetables like broccoli, carrots, and peppers. These are packed with vitamins and fiber, keeping your child feeling full without sugar spikes.
- **Go Whole Grain:** Swap white bread, pasta, and rice for whole-wheat options. These release glucose slower, preventing blood sugar spikes.
- **Lean Protein Power:** Include lean protein sources like grilled chicken, fish, or beans in every meal. Protein helps with growth and keeps you feeling satisfied.

- **Fruit in Moderation:** While fruits are good, they contain natural sugars. Choose whole fruits and limit fruit juices.
- **Limit Sugary Drinks and Processed Foods:** These are loaded with hidden sugars and unhealthy fats, wreaking havoc on blood sugar levels.

Beyond Food: Tips for Management

Healthy eating is a cornerstone, but there's more to managing type 2 diabetes:

- **Get Moving:** Encourage daily physical activity. It helps the body use glucose effectively and promotes weight management.
- **Teamwork Makes the Dream Work:** Create a personalized plan for diet, activity, and medication (if needed).
- **Open Communication:** Talk openly with your child about their diabetes. Empower them to understand their condition and be part of the management process.

Remember, a type 2 diabetes diagnosis doesn't have to define your child's life. With a healthy lifestyle and a positive attitude, your child can thrive.

Chapter 1: 30-Day Meal Plan

Week 1:

Day 1:

- Breakfast: Whole Grain Pancakes with Fresh Berries
- Lunch: Grilled Chicken Salad with Balsamic Vinaigrette
- Dinner: Baked Salmon with Asparagus
- Snack: Celery Sticks with Peanut Butter
- Dessert: Berry Yogurt Popsicles

Day 2:

- Breakfast: Veggie Egg Muffins
- Lunch: Turkey and Hummus Wrap with Veggies
- Dinner: Turkey Meatballs with Whole Wheat Pasta
- Snack: Guacamole with Carrot Sticks
- Dessert: Dark Chocolate Covered Strawberries

Day 3:

- Breakfast: Oatmeal with Apples and Cinnamon
- Lunch: Quinoa Salad with Roasted Vegetables

- Dinner: Chicken Stir-Fry with Brown Rice

- Snack: Greek Yogurt with Berries

- Dessert: Baked Apple Chips

Day 4:

- Breakfast: Greek Yogurt Parfait with Nuts and Seeds

- Lunch: Lentil Soup with Whole Grain Bread

- Dinner: Veggie and Lentil Curry

- Snack: Cottage Cheese and Pineapple

- Dessert: Frozen Banana Bites

Day 5:

- Breakfast: Spinach and Cheese Omelette

- Lunch: Tuna Salad Lettuce Wraps

- Dinner: Grilled Vegetable and Quinoa Stuffed Peppers

- Snack: Hummus and Whole Wheat Pita Chips

- Dessert: Greek Yogurt Bark with Fruit and Nuts

Day 6:

- Breakfast: Breakfast Burrito with Black Beans and Avocado

- Lunch: Veggie Stir-Fry with Tofu
- Dinner: Lemon Herb Grilled Chicken with Roasted Vegetables
- Snack: Trail Mix with Nuts and Seeds
- Dessert: Chocolate Avocado Mousse

Day 7:

- Breakfast: Chia Seed Pudding with Mixed Fruit
- Lunch: Turkey and Cheese Roll-Ups
- Dinner: Shrimp and Vegetable Skewers with Quinoa
- Snack: Apple Slices with Almond Butter
- Dessert: Rice Cake with Almond Butter and Banana Slices

Week 2:

Day 8:

- Breakfast: Quinoa Breakfast Bowl with Almonds and Honey
- Lunch: Black Bean and Corn Salad
- Dinner: Zucchini Noodles with Turkey Bolognese
- Snack: Edamame with Sea Salt
- Dessert: Baked Pear with Cinnamon

Day 9:

- Breakfast: Banana Walnut Muffins
- Lunch: Chicken and Vegetable Skewers
- Dinner: Teriyaki Tofu with Steamed Broccoli
- Snack: Veggie Sticks with Greek Yogurt Dip
- Dessert: Oatmeal Raisin Cookies with Whole Grains

Day 10:

- Breakfast: Smoothie Bowl with Spinach and Mango
- Lunch: Whole Wheat Pita Pizza with Veggies
- Dinner: Stuffed Portobello Mushrooms with Spinach and Cheese
- Snack: Baked Sweet Potato Fries
- Dessert: Pumpkin Pie Smoothie

Day 11:

- Breakfast: Whole Wheat French Toast Sticks
- Lunch: Cauliflower Fried Rice with Shrimp
- Dinner: Baked Cod with Green Beans
- Snack: Cherry Tomatoes with Mozzarella Balls
- Dessert: Coconut Chia Seed Pudding

Day 12:

- Breakfast: Breakfast Quesadilla with Turkey and Cheese
- Lunch: Greek Couscous Salad with Feta
- Dinner: Eggplant Parmesan with Whole Wheat Spaghetti
- Snack: Almonds and Dried Fruit
- Dessert: Peach and Berry Cobbler with Oat Topping

Day 13:

- Breakfast: Avocado Toast with Poached Egg
- Lunch: Turkey Chili with Beans
- Dinner: Chicken and Vegetable Kebabs with Brown Rice
- Snack: Whole Grain Crackers with Cheese
- Dessert: Mango Sorbet with Fresh Mint

Day 14:

- Breakfast: Berry Blast Smoothie with Protein Powder
- Lunch: Veggie and Bean Burrito Bowl

- Dinner: Turkey and Vegetable Stir-Fry with Cauliflower Rice
- Snack: Hard-Boiled Eggs
- Dessert: Strawberry Banana Frozen Yogurt

Week 3:

Day 15:

- Breakfast: Breakfast Wrap with Turkey Sausage and Veggies
- Lunch: Stuffed Bell Peppers with Lean Ground Beef
- Dinner: Baked Salmon with Asparagus
- Snack: Celery Sticks with Peanut Butter
- Dessert: Berry Yogurt Popsicles

Day 16:

- Breakfast: Veggie Egg Muffins
- Lunch: Turkey and Hummus Wrap with Veggies
- Dinner: Turkey Meatballs with Whole Wheat Pasta
- Snack: Guacamole with Carrot Sticks
- Dessert: Dark Chocolate Covered Strawberries

Day 17:

- Breakfast: Oatmeal with Apples and Cinnamon
- Lunch: Quinoa Salad with Roasted Vegetables
- Dinner: Chicken Stir-Fry with Brown Rice
- Snack: Greek Yogurt with Berries
- Dessert: Baked Apple Chips

Day 18:

- Breakfast: Greek Yogurt Parfait with Nuts and Seeds
- Lunch: Lentil Soup with Whole Grain Bread
- Dinner: Veggie and Lentil Curry
- Snack: Cottage Cheese and Pineapple
- Dessert: Frozen Banana Bites

Day 19:

- Breakfast: Spinach and Cheese Omelette
- Lunch: Tuna Salad Lettuce Wraps
- Dinner: Grilled Vegetable and Quinoa Stuffed Peppers
- Snack: Hummus and Whole Wheat Pita Chips
- Dessert: Greek Yogurt Bark with Fruit and Nuts

Day 20:

- Breakfast: Breakfast Burrito with Black Beans and Avocado
- Lunch: Veggie Stir-Fry with Tofu
- Dinner: Lemon Herb Grilled Chicken with Roasted Vegetables
- Snack: Trail Mix with Nuts and Seeds
- Dessert: Chocolate Avocado Mousse

Day 21:

- Breakfast: Chia Seed Pudding with Mixed Fruit
- Lunch: Turkey and Cheese Roll-Ups
- Dinner: Shrimp and Vegetable Skewers with Quinoa
- Snack: Apple Slices with Almond Butter
- Dessert: Rice Cake with Almond Butter and Banana Slices

Week 4:

Day 22:

- Breakfast: Quinoa Breakfast Bowl with Almonds and Honey
- Lunch: Black Bean and Corn Salad

- Dinner: Zucchini Noodles with Turkey Bolognese

- Snack: Edamame with Sea Salt

- Dessert: Baked Pear with Cinnamon

Day 23:

- Breakfast: Banana Walnut Muffins

- Lunch: Chicken and Vegetable Skewers

- Dinner: Teriyaki Tofu with Steamed Broccoli

- Snack: Veggie Sticks with Greek Yogurt Dip

- Dessert: Oatmeal Raisin Cookies with Whole Grains

Day 24:

- Breakfast: Smoothie Bowl with Spinach and Mango

- Lunch: Whole Wheat Pita Pizza with Veggies

- Dinner: Stuffed Portobello Mushrooms with Spinach and Cheese

- Snack: Baked Sweet Potato Fries

- Dessert: Pumpkin Pie Smoothie

Day 25:

- Breakfast: Whole Wheat French Toast Sticks

- Lunch: Cauliflower Fried Rice with Shrimp

- Dinner: Baked Cod with Green Beans

- Snack: Cherry Tomatoes with Mozzarella Balls

- Dessert: Coconut Chia Seed Pudding

Day 26:

- Breakfast: Breakfast Quesadilla with Turkey and Cheese

- Lunch: Greek Couscous Salad with Feta

- Dinner: Eggplant Parmesan with Whole Wheat Spaghetti

- Snack: Almonds and Dried Fruit

- Dessert: Peach and Berry Cobbler with Oat Topping

Day 27:

- Breakfast: Avocado Toast with Poached Egg

- Lunch: Turkey Chili with Beans

- Dinner: Chicken and Vegetable Kebabs with Brown Rice

- Snack: Whole Grain Crackers with Cheese

- Dessert: Mango Sorbet with Fresh Mint

Day 28:

- Breakfast: Berry Blast Smoothie with Protein Powder
- Lunch: Veggie and Bean Burrito Bowl
- Dinner: Turkey and Vegetable Stir-Fry with Cauliflower Rice
- Snack: Hard-Boiled Eggs
- Dessert: Strawberry Banana Frozen Yogurt

Day 29:

- Breakfast: Breakfast Wrap with Turkey Sausage and Veggies
- Lunch: Stuffed Bell Peppers with Lean Ground Beef
- Dinner: Baked Salmon with Asparagus
- Snack: Celery Sticks with Peanut Butter
- Dessert: Berry Yogurt Popsicles

Day 30:

- Breakfast: Veggie Egg Muffins
- Lunch: Turkey and Hummus Wrap with Veggies
- Dinner: Turkey Meatballs with Whole Wheat Pasta
- Snack: Guacamole with Carrot Sticks
- Dessert: Dark Chocolate Covered Strawberries

Chapter 2: Breakfast Recipes

This chapter offers a variety of delicious and balanced breakfast options that will keep energy levels stable and blood sugar in check. Each recipe is carefully crafted with wholesome ingredients and includes important nutrition information to help guide portion sizes and make informed choices.

Whole Grain Pancakes with Fresh Berries

Ingredients:

- 1 cup whole wheat flour
- 1 tablespoon baking powder
- 1 tablespoon honey
- 1 egg
- 1 cup milk (or dairy-free alternative)
- Fresh berries for topping

Instructions:

1. In a mixing bowl, combine the whole wheat flour and baking powder.
2. In a separate bowl, whisk together the honey, egg, and milk.
3. Pour the wet ingredients into the dry ingredients and stir until just combined.
4. Heat a non-stick skillet over medium heat and pour batter onto the skillet to form pancakes.
5. Cook until bubbles form on the surface, then flip and cook until golden brown on both sides.
6. Serve topped with fresh berries.

Nutrition Information:

- Calories: 200
- Protein: 8g
- Carbohydrates: 35g
- Fat: 4g
- Fiber: 5g
- Sugar: 8g
- Portion Size: 2 pancakes

Veggie Egg Muffins

Ingredients:

- 6 eggs
- 1/2 cup diced bell peppers
- 1/2 cup diced tomatoes
- 1/4 cup chopped spinach
- Salt and pepper to taste

Instructions:

1. Preheat the oven to 350°F (175°C) and grease a muffin tin.
2. In a mixing bowl, beat the eggs and season with salt and pepper.
3. Stir in the diced bell peppers, tomatoes, and chopped spinach.
4. Pour the egg mixture into the muffin tin, filling each cup about 3/4 full.
5. Bake for 20-25 minutes, or until the egg muffins are set and lightly golden.
6. Allow to cool slightly before serving.

Nutrition Information:

- Calories: 90
- Protein: 7g
- Carbohydrates: 3g
- Fat: 6g
- Fiber: 1g
- Sugar: 2g
- Portion Size: 2 egg muffins

Oatmeal with Apples and Cinnamon

Ingredients:

- 1/2 cup rolled oats
- 1 cup water
- 1/2 apple, diced
- 1/2 teaspoon cinnamon
- 1 tablespoon chopped nuts (optional)

Instructions:

1. In a small saucepan, bring the water to a boil.
2. Stir in the rolled oats and reduce heat to low.
3. Cook for 5-7 minutes, stirring occasionally, until the oats are tender.

4. Stir in the diced apple and cinnamon.

5. Cook for an additional 2-3 minutes, until the apple is soft.

6. Serve hot, topped with chopped nuts if desired.

Nutrition Information:

- Calories: 150

- Protein: 5g

- Carbohydrates: 27g

- Fat: 3g

- Fiber: 5g

- Sugar: 9g

- Portion Size: 1 cup

Greek Yogurt Parfait with Nuts and Seeds

Ingredients:

- 1/2 cup Greek yogurt

- 1/4 cup mixed nuts and seeds (such as almonds, walnuts, pumpkin seeds, and sunflower seeds)

- 1/4 cup mixed berries (such as strawberries, blueberries, and raspberries)
- 1 tablespoon honey (optional)

Instructions:

1. In a glass or bowl, layer the Greek yogurt, mixed nuts and seeds, and mixed berries.
2. Drizzle honey on top if desired.
3. Repeat the layers until ingredients are used up.
4. Serve chilled.

Nutrition Information:

- Calories: 250
- Protein: 15g
- Carbohydrates: 20g
- Fat: 12g
- Fiber: 5g
- Sugar: 10g
- Portion Size: 1 serving

Spinach and Cheese Omelette

Ingredients:

- 2 eggs
- 1/4 cup chopped spinach
- 1/4 cup shredded cheese
- Salt and pepper to taste

Instructions:

1. In a bowl, beat the eggs and season with salt and pepper.
2. Heat a non-stick skillet over medium heat and pour in the beaten eggs.
3. Cook until the edges begin to set, then sprinkle the chopped spinach and shredded cheese over one half of the omelette.
4. Fold the other half of the omelette over the filling and cook for another minute or until the cheese is melted.
5. Slide the omelette onto a plate and serve hot.

Nutrition Information:

- Calories: 220
- Protein: 17g

- Carbohydrates: 2g
- Fat: 16g
- Fiber: 1g
- Sugar: 1g
- Portion Size: 1 omelette

Breakfast Burrito with Black Beans and Avocado

Ingredients:

- 1 whole wheat tortilla
- 1/4 cup black beans, drained and rinsed
- 1/4 avocado, sliced
- 2 tablespoons salsa
- 1 egg, scrambled

Instructions:

1. Heat the whole wheat tortilla in a skillet or microwave until warm.
2. Layer the black beans, sliced avocado, salsa, and scrambled egg onto the tortilla.
3. Roll up the tortilla to form a burrito.

4. Serve immediately.

Nutrition Information:

- Calories: 300
- Protein: 14g
- Carbohydrates: 30g
- Fat: 15g
- Fiber: 9g
- Sugar: 2g
- Portion Size: 1 burrito

Chia Seed Pudding with Mixed Fruit

Ingredients:

- 2 tablespoons chia seeds
- 1/2 cup milk (or dairy-free alternative)
- 1/2 teaspoon vanilla extract
- Mixed fruit for topping (such as berries, kiwi, and mango)

Instructions:

1. In a bowl, mix together the chia seeds, milk, and vanilla extract.

2. Refrigerate for at least 2 hours or overnight, until the chia seeds have absorbed the liquid and the mixture has thickened.

3. Stir the chia seed pudding before serving and top with mixed fruit.

Nutrition Information:

- Calories: 180
- Protein: 5g
- Carbohydrates: 20g
- Fat: 8g
- Fiber: 8g
- Sugar: 10g
- Portion Size: 1 serving

Quinoa Breakfast Bowl with Almonds and Honey

Ingredients:

- 1/2 cup cooked quinoa
- 1 tablespoon almonds, sliced
- 1 tablespoon honey

- 1/4 teaspoon cinnamon

Instructions:

1. In a bowl, layer the cooked quinoa.
2. Top with sliced almonds, drizzle with honey, and sprinkle with cinnamon.
3. Serve warm.

Nutrition Information:

- Calories: 220
- Protein: 6g
- Carbohydrates: 35g
- Fat: 6g
- Fiber: 4g
- Sugar: 10g
- Portion Size: 1 serving

Banana Walnut Muffins

Ingredients:

- 1 cup whole wheat flour
- 1/2 cup mashed ripe banana
- 1/4 cup chopped walnuts

- 1/4 cup honey
- 1/4 cup Greek yogurt
- 1 egg
- 1 teaspoon baking powder
- 1/2 teaspoon cinnamon

Instructions:

1. Preheat the oven to 350°F (175°C) and line a muffin tin with liners.
2. In a mixing bowl, combine the whole wheat flour, mashed banana, chopped walnuts, honey, Greek yogurt, egg, baking powder, and cinnamon.
3. Stir until just combined.
4. Divide the batter evenly among the muffin cups.
5. Bake for 20-25 minutes, or until a toothpick inserted into the center comes out clean.
6. Allow the muffins to cool before serving.

Nutrition Information:

- Calories: 150
- Protein: 5g
- Carbohydrates: 25g

- Fat: 5g

- Fiber: 3g

- Sugar: 10g

- Portion Size: 1 muffin

Smoothie Bowl with Spinach and Mango

Ingredients:

- 1 cup frozen mango chunks

- 1/2 cup spinach

- 1/2 cup Greek yogurt

- 1/4 cup almond milk

- 1 tablespoon honey

- Toppings: sliced banana, granola, shredded coconut

Instructions:

1. In a blender, combine the frozen mango chunks, spinach, Greek yogurt, almond milk, and honey.

2. Blend until smooth and creamy.

3. Pour the smoothie into a bowl.

4. Top with sliced banana, granola, and shredded coconut.

5. Serve immediately.

Nutrition Information:

- Calories: 250

- Protein: 10g

- Carbohydrates: 40g

- Fat: 6g

- Fiber: 5g

- Sugar: 30g

- Portion Size: 1 serving

Whole Wheat French Toast Sticks

Ingredients:

- 2 slices whole wheat bread

- 1 egg

- 1/4 cup milk (or dairy-free alternative)

- 1/2 teaspoon vanilla extract

- 1/4 teaspoon cinnamon

- Cooking spray

Instructions:

1. Cut the whole wheat bread into sticks.
2. In a shallow bowl, whisk together the egg, milk, vanilla extract, and cinnamon.
3. Dip each bread stick into the egg mixture, coating evenly.
4. Heat a non-stick skillet over medium heat and lightly coat with cooking spray.
5. Cook the French toast sticks for 2-3 minutes on each side, or until golden brown.
6. Serve warm with a drizzle of maple syrup if desired.

Nutrition Information:

- Calories: 180
- Protein: 8g
- Carbohydrates: 25g
- Fat: 5g
- Fiber: 3g
- Sugar: 5g
- Portion Size: 4 sticks

Breakfast Quesadilla with Turkey and Cheese

Ingredients:

- 1 whole wheat tortilla
- 2 slices turkey breast
- 1/4 cup shredded cheese
- 1/4 avocado, sliced
- Salsa for dipping

Instructions:

1. Heat a non-stick skillet over medium heat.
2. Place the whole wheat tortilla in the skillet and top with turkey slices, shredded cheese, and avocado slices.
3. Fold the tortilla in half and cook for 2-3 minutes on each side, or until the cheese is melted and the tortilla is golden brown.
4. Cut the quesadilla into wedges and serve with salsa for dipping.

Nutrition Information:

- Calories: 280

- Protein: 18g

- Carbohydrates: 20g

- Fat: 14g

- Fiber: 5g

- Sugar: 2g

- Portion Size: 1 quesadilla

Avocado Toast with Poached Egg

Ingredients:

- 1 slice whole wheat bread

- 1/2 avocado, mashed

- 1 egg

- Salt and pepper to taste

Instructions:

1. Toast the whole wheat bread until golden brown.

2. Spread the mashed avocado onto the toast and sprinkle with salt and pepper.

3. Fill a saucepan with water and bring to a gentle simmer.

4. Crack the egg into a small bowl, then carefully slide it into the simmering water.

5. Cook for 3-4 minutes, until the egg white is set but the yolk is still runny.
6. Remove the poached egg with a slotted spoon and place it on top of the avocado toast.
7. Serve immediately.

Nutrition Information:

- Calories: 220
- Protein: 10g
- Carbohydrates: 15g
- Fat: 14g
- Fiber: 7g
- Sugar: 1g
- Portion Size: 1 serving

Berry Blast Smoothie with Protein Powder

Ingredients:

- 1/2 cup mixed berries (such as strawberries, blueberries, and raspberries)
- 1/2 banana, sliced

- 1/2 cup Greek yogurt
- 1/2 cup almond milk
- 1 scoop protein powder (vanilla or berry flavored)

Instructions:

1. In a blender, combine the mixed berries, sliced banana, Greek yogurt, almond milk, and protein powder.
2. Blend until smooth and creamy.
3. Pour into a glass and serve immediately.

Nutrition Information:

- Calories: 250
- Protein: 20g
- Carbohydrates: 30g
- Fat: 5g
- Fiber: 7g
- Sugar: 15g
- Portion Size: 1 serving

Breakfast Wrap with Turkey Sausage and Veggies

Ingredients:

- 1 whole wheat tortilla
- 1 turkey sausage patty, cooked and crumbled
- 1/4 cup diced bell peppers
- 1/4 cup diced tomatoes
- 1/4 cup shredded cheese
- Salsa for dipping

Instructions:

1. Heat the whole wheat tortilla in a skillet until warm.
2. Layer the cooked turkey sausage, diced bell peppers, diced tomatoes, and shredded cheese onto the tortilla.
3. Roll up the tortilla to form a wrap.
4. Slice in half and serve with salsa for dipping.

Nutrition Information:

- Calories: 300
- Protein: 18g
- Carbohydrates: 20g
- Fat: 15g

- Fiber: 5g

- Sugar: 2g

- Portion Size: 1 wrap

These recipes are designed to provide balanced nutrition while offering exciting flavors and textures to keep kids satisfied and energized throughout the day. From hearty salads to flavorful wraps and comforting soups, each recipe is crafted with wholesome ingredients and simple instructions to make mealtime both nutritious and enjoyable for your little ones.

Grilled Chicken Salad with Balsamic Vinaigrette

Ingredients:

- 2 boneless, skinless chicken breasts
- 6 cups mixed salad greens
- 1 cup cherry tomatoes, halved
- 1/2 cucumber, sliced
- 1/4 red onion, thinly sliced
- 1/4 cup balsamic vinegar
- 2 tablespoons olive oil
- Salt and pepper to taste

Instructions:

1. Preheat grill to medium-high heat.
2. Season chicken breasts with salt and pepper.
3. Grill chicken for 6-8 minutes per side or until cooked through.
4. In a small bowl, whisk together balsamic vinegar, olive oil, salt, and pepper to make the vinaigrette.
5. In a large bowl, toss salad greens, cherry tomatoes, cucumber, and red onion with the balsamic vinaigrette.
6. Slice grilled chicken and arrange on top of the salad.
7. Serve immediately.

Nutrition Information:

- Calories: 320
- Protein: 28g
- Carbohydrates: 10g
- Fat: 18g
- Fiber: 4g
- Sugar: 5g
- Portion Size: 1 serving

Turkey and Hummus Wrap with Veggies

Ingredients:

- 4 whole wheat tortillas
- 1 cup hummus
- 8 slices turkey breast
- 1 cup mixed salad greens
- 1/2 red bell pepper, thinly sliced
- 1/2 yellow bell pepper, thinly sliced
- 1/2 cup shredded carrots

Instructions:

1. Spread hummus evenly on each tortilla.
2. Layer turkey slices, salad greens, bell peppers, and shredded carrots on top of the hummus.
3. Roll up tortillas tightly, tucking in the sides as you go.
4. Slice wraps in half diagonally and serve.

Nutrition Information:

- Calories: 280
- Protein: 20g

- Carbohydrates: 30g

- Fat: 10g

- Fiber: 8g

- Sugar: 3g

- Portion Size: 1 wrap

Quinoa Salad with Roasted Vegetables

Ingredients:

- 1 cup quinoa, rinsed

- 2 cups water or vegetable broth

- 2 cups mixed vegetables (such as bell peppers, zucchini, and cherry tomatoes), chopped

- 2 tablespoons olive oil

- Salt and pepper to taste

- 1/4 cup feta cheese, crumbled

- 2 tablespoons fresh parsley, chopped

Instructions:

1. Preheat oven to 400°F (200°C).

2. In a saucepan, bring water or vegetable broth to a
   boil. Add quinoa, reduce heat to low, cover, and
   simmer for 15 minutes or until quinoa is cooked and
   water is absorbed.

3. Meanwhile, toss mixed vegetables with olive oil,
   salt, and pepper on a baking sheet.

4. Roast vegetables in the preheated oven for 20-25
   minutes or until tender and slightly browned.

5. In a large bowl, combine cooked quinoa, roasted
   vegetables, feta cheese, and fresh parsley. Toss
   gently to mix.

6. Serve warm or chilled.

Nutrition Information:

- Calories: 280
- Protein: 8g
- Carbohydrates: 35g
- Fat: 12g
- Fiber: 6g
- Sugar: 4g
- Portion Size: 1 cup

Lentil Soup with Whole Grain Bread

Ingredients:

- 1 cup dried green lentils, rinsed
- 4 cups vegetable broth
- 1 onion, diced
- 2 carrots, diced
- 2 celery stalks, diced
- 2 cloves garlic, minced
- 1 teaspoon ground cumin
- 1 teaspoon smoked paprika
- Salt and pepper to taste
- 4 slices whole grain bread, toasted

Instructions:

1. In a large pot, combine lentils, vegetable broth, onion, carrots, celery, garlic, cumin, and smoked paprika.
2. Bring the mixture to a boil, then reduce heat to low and simmer for 25-30 minutes or until lentils and vegetables are tender.
3. Season with salt and pepper to taste.

4. Ladle soup into bowls and serve with toasted whole grain bread on the side.

Nutrition Information:

- Calories: 250
- Protein: 15g
- Carbohydrates: 45g
- Fat: 2g
- Fiber: 15g
- Sugar: 5g
- Portion Size: 1.5 cups soup with 1 slice of bread

Tuna Salad Lettuce Wraps

Ingredients:

- 2 cans (5 oz each) tuna, drained
- 1/4 cup Greek yogurt
- 2 tablespoons lemon juice
- 1/4 cup diced red onion
- 1/4 cup diced celery
- 1/4 cup diced red bell pepper
- Salt and pepper to taste
- 8 large lettuce leaves

Instructions:

1. In a bowl, combine tuna, Greek yogurt, lemon juice, red onion, celery, and red bell pepper. Mix well.
2. Season with salt and pepper to taste.
3. Place a scoop of tuna salad onto each lettuce leaf.
4. Roll up lettuce leaves and secure with toothpicks if needed.
5. Serve chilled.

Nutrition Information:

- Calories: 180
- Protein: 25g
- Carbohydrates: 6g
- Fat: 5g
- Fiber: 2g
- Sugar: 2g
- Portion Size: 2 lettuce wraps

Veggie Stir-Fry with Tofu

Ingredients:

- 14 oz firm tofu, drained and cubed
- 2 tablespoons soy sauce

- 1 tablespoon sesame oil

- 2 cloves garlic, minced

- 1 teaspoon ginger, minced

- 2 cups mixed vegetables (such as bell peppers, broccoli, and snap peas), sliced

- Cooked brown rice for serving

Instructions:

1. In a bowl, marinate tofu cubes in soy sauce for 15-20 minutes.

2. Heat sesame oil in a large skillet or wok over medium-high heat.

3. Add garlic and ginger, and sauté for 1 minute.

4. Add marinated tofu cubes and cook until golden brown on all sides.

5. Add mixed vegetables to the skillet and stir-fry until tender-crisp.

6. Serve stir-fried tofu and vegetables over cooked brown rice.

Nutrition Information:

- Calories: 280

- Protein: 20g

- Carbohydrates: 25g

- Fat: 12g

- Fiber: 6g

- Sugar: 5g

- Portion Size: 1 cup stir-fry with 1/2 cup brown rice

Turkey and Cheese Roll-Ups

Ingredients:

- 4 slices deli turkey breast

- 4 slices reduced-fat cheese (such as cheddar or Swiss)

- 1/2 cucumber, cut into thin strips

- 1/2 red bell pepper, cut into thin strips

- 1/2 yellow bell pepper, cut into thin strips

Instructions:

1. Lay out turkey slices on a clean surface.

2. Place a slice of cheese on top of each turkey slice.

3. Arrange cucumber and bell pepper strips on one end of each turkey slice.

4. Roll up turkey slices tightly, enclosing the vegetables.

5. Secure roll-ups with toothpicks if needed.

6. Slice each roll-up into bite-sized pieces and serve.

Nutrition Information:

- Calories: 180

- Protein: 15g

- Carbohydrates: 5g

- Fat: 10g

- Fiber: 1g

- Sugar: 3g

- Portion Size: 2 roll-ups

Black Bean and Corn Salad

Ingredients:

- 1 can (15 oz) black beans, drained and rinsed

- 1 cup frozen corn kernels, thawed

- 1/4 cup red onion, finely chopped

- 1/4 cup fresh cilantro, chopped

- 1 avocado, diced

- 2 tablespoons lime juice

- 1 tablespoon olive oil
- Salt and pepper to taste

Instructions:

1. In a large bowl, combine black beans, corn, red onion, cilantro, and avocado.
2. Drizzle lime juice and olive oil over the salad.
3. Season with salt and pepper to taste.
4. Toss gently to mix all ingredients together.
5. Serve chilled or at room temperature.

Nutrition Information:

- Calories: 220
- Protein: 8g
- Carbohydrates: 30g
- Fat: 9g
- Fiber: 10g
- Sugar: 2g
- Portion Size: 1 cup salad

Chicken and Vegetable Skewers

Ingredients:

- 2 boneless, skinless chicken breasts, cut into cubes
- 1 zucchini, sliced
- 1 yellow bell pepper, cut into chunks
- 1 red onion, cut into chunks
- 8 cherry tomatoes
- 2 tablespoons olive oil
- 2 tablespoons balsamic vinegar
- 1 teaspoon Italian seasoning
- Salt and pepper to taste

Instructions:

1. Preheat grill to medium-high heat.
2. Thread chicken cubes and vegetables onto skewers, alternating between chicken and vegetables.
3. In a small bowl, whisk together olive oil, balsamic vinegar, Italian seasoning, salt, and pepper to make the marinade.
4. Brush marinade over skewers, coating evenly.

5. Grill skewers for 8-10 minutes, turning occasionally, until chicken is cooked through and vegetables are tender.

6. Serve hot off the grill.

Nutrition Information:

- Calories: 280
- Protein: 25g
- Carbohydrates: 15g
- Fat: 12g
- Fiber: 4g
- Sugar: 6g
- Portion Size: 2 skewers

Whole Wheat Pita Pizza with Veggies

Ingredients:

- 4 whole wheat pita bread rounds
- 1/2 cup pizza sauce
- 1 cup shredded part-skim mozzarella cheese

- 1 cup assorted vegetables (such as bell peppers, mushrooms, and onions), sliced
- 1 tablespoon olive oil
- 1 teaspoon Italian seasoning

Instructions:

1. Preheat oven to 400°F (200°C).
2. Place whole wheat pita bread rounds on a baking sheet.
3. Spread pizza sauce evenly over each pita bread round.
4. Sprinkle shredded mozzarella cheese over the sauce.
5. Arrange sliced vegetables on top of the cheese.
6. Drizzle olive oil over the vegetables and sprinkle with Italian seasoning.
7. Bake in the preheated oven for 10-12 minutes or until cheese is melted and bubbly.
8. Slice each whole wheat pita pizza into wedges and serve.

Nutrition Information:

- Calories: 220

- Protein: 12g

- Carbohydrates: 30g

- Fat: 8g

- Fiber: 6g

- Sugar: 4g

- Portion Size: 1 whole wheat pita pizza

Cauliflower Fried Rice with Shrimp

Ingredients:

- 1 head cauliflower, grated

- 1 tablespoon sesame oil

- 1 onion, diced

- 2 cloves garlic, minced

- 1 cup mixed vegetables (such as peas, carrots, and corn)

- 8 oz shrimp, peeled and deveined

- 2 tablespoons soy sauce

- 2 eggs, beaten

- Green onions for garnish

Instructions:

1. In a large skillet or wok, heat sesame oil over medium heat.
2. Add diced onion and minced garlic, and sauté until fragrant.
3. Stir in mixed vegetables and cook until tender.
4. Add grated cauliflower to the skillet and stir-fry until cauliflower is tender.
5. Push cauliflower mixture to one side of the skillet and add beaten eggs to the other side.
6. Scramble eggs until cooked through, then mix with the cauliflower mixture.
7. Stir in shrimp and soy sauce, and cook until shrimp are pink and cooked through.
8. Garnish with chopped green onions before serving.

Nutrition Information:

- Calories: 250
- Protein: 20g
- Carbohydrates: 20g
- Fat: 10g
- Fiber: 6g

- Sugar: 6g

- Portion Size: 1.5 cups

Greek Couscous Salad with Feta

Ingredients:

- 1 cup whole wheat couscous, cooked

- 1 cup cherry tomatoes, halved

- 1 cucumber, diced

- 1/4 cup red onion, thinly sliced

- 1/4 cup Kalamata olives, pitted and sliced

- 1/4 cup crumbled feta cheese

- 2 tablespoons fresh lemon juice

- 2 tablespoons extra virgin olive oil

- 1 tablespoon fresh oregano, chopped

- Salt and pepper to taste

Instructions:

1. In a large bowl, combine cooked couscous, cherry tomatoes, cucumber, red onion, Kalamata olives, and feta cheese.

2. In a small bowl, whisk together lemon juice, olive oil, fresh oregano, salt, and pepper to make the dressing.

3. Pour dressing over the salad and toss gently to coat all ingredients.

4. Serve chilled or at room temperature.

Nutrition Information:

- Calories: 280
- Protein: 10g
- Carbohydrates: 35g
- Fat: 12g
- Fiber: 6g
- Sugar: 4g
- Portion Size: 1 cup salad

Turkey Chili with Beans

Ingredients:

- 1 tablespoon olive oil
- 1 onion, diced
- 2 cloves garlic, minced
- 1 lb lean ground turkey

- 1 can (15 oz) kidney beans, drained and rinsed

- 1 can (15 oz) black beans, drained and rinsed

- 1 can (14.5 oz) diced tomatoes

- 1 cup low-sodium chicken broth

- 1 tablespoon chili powder

- 1 teaspoon ground cumin

- 1/2 teaspoon paprika

- Salt and pepper to taste

- Optional toppings: shredded cheese, Greek yogurt, chopped green onions

Instructions:

1. Heat olive oil in a large pot over medium heat.

2. Add diced onion and minced garlic, and sauté until softened.

3. Add ground turkey to the pot and cook until browned, breaking it up with a spoon.

4. Stir in kidney beans, black beans, diced tomatoes, chicken broth, chili powder, cumin, paprika, salt, and pepper.

5. Bring the chili to a simmer, then reduce heat to low and let it cook for 20-25 minutes, stirring occasionally.
6. Adjust seasoning to taste, if needed.
7. Serve hot, topped with optional toppings if desired.

Nutrition Information:

- Calories: 280
- Protein: 25g
- Carbohydrates: 30g
- Fat: 8g
- Fiber: 10g
- Sugar: 5g
- Portion Size: 1.5 cups

Veggie and Bean Burrito Bowl

Ingredients:

- 1 cup cooked brown rice
- 1 cup canned black beans, drained and rinsed
- 1 cup corn kernels (fresh, frozen, or canned)
- 1 bell pepper, diced
- 1 avocado, diced

- 1/4 cup salsa
- 1/4 cup plain Greek yogurt (or sour cream)
- Fresh cilantro for garnish

Instructions:

1. Divide cooked brown rice evenly among serving bowls.
2. Top each bowl with black beans, corn kernels, diced bell pepper, diced avocado, salsa, and Greek yogurt.
3. Garnish with fresh cilantro.
4. Serve immediately.

Nutrition Information:

- Calories: 320
- Protein: 12g
- Carbohydrates: 45g
- Fat: 10g
- Fiber: 12g
- Sugar: 5g
- Portion Size: 1 bowl

Stuffed Bell Peppers with Lean Ground Beef

Ingredients:

- 4 bell peppers, any color
- 1 lb lean ground beef
- 1 onion, diced
- 2 cloves garlic, minced
- 1 cup cooked quinoa
- 1 can (14.5 oz) diced tomatoes, drained
- 1 cup shredded reduced-fat cheese
- 1 teaspoon Italian seasoning
- Salt and pepper to taste

Instructions:

1. Preheat oven to 375°F (190°C).
2. Cut the tops off the bell peppers and remove seeds and membranes.
3. In a large skillet, cook ground beef, onion, and garlic over medium heat until beef is browned and onion is softened.
4. Stir in cooked quinoa, diced tomatoes, Italian seasoning, salt, and pepper.

5. Spoon beef mixture into each bell pepper until filled.

6. Place stuffed bell peppers in a baking dish and cover with foil.

7. Bake in the preheated oven for 30-35 minutes or until peppers are tender.

8. Remove foil, sprinkle shredded cheese over the tops of the peppers, and bake for an additional 5 minutes until cheese is melted.

9. Serve hot.

Nutrition Information:

- Calories: 320
- Protein: 25g
- Carbohydrates: 25g
- Fat: 12g
- Fiber: 6g
- Sugar: 8g
- Portion Size: 1 stuffed bell pepper

Chapter 4: Dinner Recipes

In this chapter, we've curated dinner recipes that are not only kid-friendly but also easy to prepare and packed with wholesome ingredients. From succulent seafood to hearty vegetarian dishes, there's something for everyone to enjoy.

Baked Salmon with Asparagus

Ingredients:

- 4 salmon fillets
- 1 bunch of asparagus, trimmed
- 2 tablespoons olive oil
- 2 cloves garlic, minced
- Salt and pepper to taste
- Lemon wedges for serving

Instructions:

1. Preheat the oven to 400°F (200°C).
2. Place the salmon fillets on a baking sheet lined with parchment paper.
3. Arrange the asparagus around the salmon.

4. Drizzle olive oil over the salmon and asparagus, then sprinkle with minced garlic, salt, and pepper.

5. Bake for 12-15 minutes, or until the salmon is cooked through and flakes easily with a fork.

6. Serve hot with lemon wedges on the side.

Nutrition Information (per serving):

- Calories: 320
- Protein: 30g
- Carbohydrates: 6g
- Fat: 20g
- Fiber: 3g
- Sugar: 2g
- Portion Size: 1 salmon fillet with asparagus

Turkey Meatballs with Whole Wheat Pasta

Ingredients:

- 1 lb lean ground turkey
- 1/2 cup whole wheat breadcrumbs
- 1/4 cup grated Parmesan cheese

- 1 egg
- 2 cloves garlic, minced
- 1 teaspoon dried oregano
- 1/2 teaspoon salt
- 1/4 teaspoon black pepper
- 2 cups cooked whole wheat pasta
- Marinara sauce (optional)

Instructions:

1. Preheat the oven to 375°F (190°C).
2. In a large bowl, combine ground turkey, breadcrumbs, Parmesan cheese, egg, minced garlic, dried oregano, salt, and pepper. Mix until well combined.
3. Shape the mixture into meatballs and place them on a baking sheet lined with parchment paper.
4. Bake for 20-25 minutes, or until the meatballs are cooked through and browned.
5. Serve the meatballs over cooked whole wheat pasta and top with marinara sauce if desired.

Nutrition Information (per serving):

- Calories: 350
- Protein: 28g
- Carbohydrates: 25g
- Fat: 14g
- Fiber: 4g
- Sugar: 2g
- Portion Size: 4 meatballs with pasta

Chicken Stir-Fry with Brown Rice

Ingredients:

- 1 lb boneless, skinless chicken breasts, sliced thinly
- 2 cups mixed vegetables (such as bell peppers, broccoli, carrots)
- 2 tablespoons low-sodium soy sauce
- 1 tablespoon olive oil
- 2 cloves garlic, minced
- 1 teaspoon ginger, grated
- Cooked brown rice for serving

Instructions:

1. Heat olive oil in a large skillet or wok over medium-high heat.
2. Add minced garlic and grated ginger, and sauté for 1 minute until fragrant.
3. Add sliced chicken to the skillet and cook until browned and cooked through.
4. Add mixed vegetables to the skillet and stir-fry for 3-4 minutes until tender-crisp.
5. Pour low-sodium soy sauce over the chicken and vegetables, and toss to coat evenly.
6. Serve hot over cooked brown rice.

Nutrition Information (per serving):

- Calories: 320
- Protein: 28g
- Carbohydrates: 30g
- Fat: 8g
- Fiber: 5g
- Sugar: 3g
- Portion Size: 1 cup of chicken stir-fry with brown rice

Veggie and Lentil Curry

Ingredients:

- 1 cup dried lentils, rinsed and drained
- 2 cups mixed vegetables (such as cauliflower, peas, carrots)
- 1 can (14 oz) coconut milk
- 2 tablespoons curry powder
- 1 tablespoon olive oil
- 1 onion, chopped
- 2 cloves garlic, minced
- Salt and pepper to taste
- Cooked brown rice for serving

Instructions:

1. Heat olive oil in a large pot over medium heat.
2. Add chopped onion and minced garlic, and sauté until softened.
3. Stir in curry powder and cook for 1 minute until fragrant.
4. Add mixed vegetables and dried lentils to the pot, then pour in coconut milk.

5. Season with salt and pepper to taste, and bring to a simmer.

6. Cover and cook for 20-25 minutes, or until lentils are tender and vegetables are cooked through.

7. Serve hot over cooked brown rice.

Nutrition Information (per serving):

- Calories: 380

- Protein: 18g

- Carbohydrates: 45g

- Fat: 16g

- Fiber: 12g

- Sugar: 6g

- Portion Size: 1 cup of curry with brown rice

Grilled Vegetable and Quinoa Stuffed Peppers

Ingredients:

- 4 large bell peppers, halved and seeds removed

- 1 cup quinoa, rinsed

- 2 cups vegetable broth

- 2 cups mixed grilled vegetables (such as zucchini, bell peppers, eggplant)
- 1 cup cherry tomatoes, halved
- 1/4 cup crumbled feta cheese (optional)
- 2 tablespoons chopped fresh basil
- Salt and pepper to taste

Instructions:

1. Preheat the grill to medium heat.
2. In a medium saucepan, bring the vegetable broth to a boil.
3. Add quinoa, reduce heat to low, cover, and simmer for 15-20 minutes, or until quinoa is cooked and liquid is absorbed.
4. In a large bowl, combine cooked quinoa, grilled vegetables, cherry tomatoes, crumbled feta cheese (if using), chopped fresh basil, salt, and pepper.
5. Fill each bell pepper half with the quinoa and vegetable mixture.
6. Grill the stuffed peppers for 10-15 minutes, or until the peppers are tender and slightly charred.

7. Serve hot, garnished with additional fresh basil if desired.

Nutrition Information (per serving):

- Calories: 280
- Protein: 9g
- Carbohydrates: 45g
- Fat: 6g
- Fiber: 8g
- Sugar: 8g
- Portion Size: 2 stuffed pepper halves

Lemon Herb Grilled Chicken with Roasted Vegetables

Ingredients:

- 4 boneless, skinless chicken breasts
- 2 tablespoons olive oil
- 2 tablespoons lemon juice
- 2 cloves garlic, minced
- 1 teaspoon dried thyme
- 1 teaspoon dried rosemary

- Salt and pepper to taste

- 4 cups mixed vegetables (such as bell peppers, zucchini, red onion)

Instructions:

1. In a small bowl, whisk together olive oil, lemon juice, minced garlic, dried thyme, dried rosemary, salt, and pepper.
2. Place chicken breasts in a shallow dish and pour the marinade over them. Marinate in the refrigerator for at least 30 minutes.
3. Preheat the grill to medium-high heat.
4. Thread mixed vegetables onto skewers and brush with olive oil.
5. Grill chicken breasts for 6-8 minutes per side, or until cooked through and no longer pink in the center.
6. Grill vegetable skewers for 8-10 minutes, or until tender and lightly charred.
7. Serve hot, with roasted vegetables alongside grilled chicken.

Nutrition Information (per serving):

- Calories: 320
- Protein: 32g
- Carbohydrates: 15g
- Fat: 14g
- Fiber: 5g
- Sugar: 5g
- Portion Size: 1 grilled chicken breast with roasted vegetables

Shrimp and Vegetable Skewers with Quinoa

Ingredients:

- 1 lb large shrimp, peeled and deveined
- 2 bell peppers, cut into chunks
- 1 red onion, cut into chunks
- 1 zucchini, sliced
- 1 cup cherry tomatoes
- 2 tablespoons olive oil
- 2 cloves garlic, minced
- 1 teaspoon dried oregano

- Salt and pepper to taste
- Cooked quinoa for serving

Instructions:

1. Preheat the grill to medium-high heat.
2. Thread shrimp, bell peppers, red onion, zucchini, and cherry tomatoes onto skewers.
3. In a small bowl, whisk together olive oil, minced garlic, dried oregano, salt, and pepper.
4. Brush the marinade over the shrimp and vegetables skewers.
5. Grill the skewers for 2-3 minutes per side, or until the shrimp are pink and opaque.
6. Serve hot over cooked quinoa.

Nutrition Information (per serving):

- Calories: 280
- Protein: 25g
- Carbohydrates: 20g
- Fat: 10g
- Fiber: 4g
- Sugar: 5g

- Portion Size: 2 skewers with quinoa

Beef and Broccoli Stir-Fry

Ingredients:

- 1 lb flank steak, thinly sliced
- 2 cups broccoli florets
- 1 bell pepper, sliced
- 1 onion, sliced
- 2 cloves garlic, minced
- 1/4 cup low-sodium soy sauce
- 2 tablespoons honey
- 1 tablespoon cornstarch
- 1 teaspoon sesame oil
- Cooked brown rice for serving

Instructions:

1. In a small bowl, whisk together low-sodium soy sauce, honey, cornstarch, and sesame oil to make the sauce.
2. Heat olive oil in a large skillet or wok over medium-high heat.

3. Add minced garlic and cook for 1 minute until fragrant.

4. Add sliced flank steak to the skillet and stir-fry until browned.

5. Add broccoli florets, bell pepper, and onion to the skillet, and stir-fry for 3-4 minutes until vegetables are tender-crisp.

6. Pour the sauce over the beef and vegetables, and toss to coat evenly.

7. Cook for an additional 2-3 minutes until the sauce has thickened.

8. Serve hot over cooked brown rice.

Nutrition Information (per serving):

- Calories: 380
- Protein: 30g
- Carbohydrates: 30g
- Fat: 15g
- Fiber: 5g
- Sugar: 10g
- Portion Size: 1 cup of beef and broccoli stir-fry with brown rice

Zucchini Noodles with Turkey Bolognese

Ingredients:

- 1 lb lean ground turkey
- 4 medium zucchini, spiralized into noodles
- 1 can (14 oz) crushed tomatoes
- 2 cloves garlic, minced
- 1 onion, chopped
- 1 carrot, grated
- 1 stalk celery, chopped
- 1 teaspoon dried oregano
- 1 teaspoon dried basil
- Salt and pepper to taste
- Grated Parmesan cheese for serving

Instructions:

1. Heat olive oil in a large skillet over medium heat.
2. Add minced garlic, chopped onion, grated carrot, and chopped celery to the skillet. Sauté until vegetables are softened.
3. Add lean ground turkey to the skillet and cook until browned.

4. Stir in crushed tomatoes, dried oregano, dried basil, salt, and pepper. Simmer for 10-15 minutes.

5. Meanwhile, spiralize zucchini into noodles using a spiralizer.

6. Add zucchini noodles to the skillet and cook for 2-3 minutes until tender.

7. Serve hot, topped with grated Parmesan cheese.

Nutrition Information (per serving):

- Calories: 290

- Protein: 26g

- Carbohydrates: 20g

- Fat: 10g

- Fiber: 6g

- Sugar: 10g

- Portion Size: 1 cup of turkey bolognese with zucchini noodles

Teriyaki Tofu with Steamed Broccoli

Ingredients:

- 1 block (14 oz) firm tofu, drained and pressed

- 1 head broccoli, cut into florets

- 1/4 cup low-sodium soy sauce

- 2 tablespoons honey

- 1 tablespoon rice vinegar

- 2 cloves garlic, minced

- 1 teaspoon grated ginger

- 1 tablespoon cornstarch

- Cooked brown rice for serving

Instructions:

1. Preheat the oven to 400°F (200°C).

2. Cut pressed tofu into cubes and place them on a baking sheet lined with parchment paper.

3. Bake tofu cubes for 25-30 minutes, or until golden brown and crispy.

4. Steam broccoli florets until tender-crisp.

5. In a small saucepan, whisk together low-sodium soy sauce, honey, rice vinegar, minced garlic, grated ginger, and cornstarch. Cook over medium heat until the sauce thickens.

6. Toss baked tofu cubes in the teriyaki sauce until coated.

7. Serve hot, with steamed broccoli and cooked brown rice.

Nutrition Information (per serving):

- Calories: 320
- Protein: 20g
- Carbohydrates: 40g
- Fat: 10g
- Fiber: 6g
- Sugar: 12g
- Portion Size: 1 cup of teriyaki tofu with steamed broccoli and brown rice

Stuffed Portobello Mushrooms with Spinach and Cheese

Ingredients:

- 4 large portobello mushrooms, stems removed
- 2 cups baby spinach, chopped
- 1/2 cup low-fat ricotta cheese
- 1/4 cup grated Parmesan cheese
- 2 cloves garlic, minced

- 1 tablespoon olive oil
- Salt and pepper to taste

Instructions:

1. Preheat the oven to 375°F (190°C).
2. Place portobello mushrooms on a baking sheet lined with parchment paper.
3. In a skillet, heat olive oil over medium heat. Add minced garlic and chopped spinach, and cook until spinach is wilted.
4. In a bowl, combine chopped spinach, ricotta cheese, grated Parmesan cheese, salt, and pepper.
5. Fill each portobello mushroom with the spinach and cheese mixture.
6. Bake stuffed mushrooms in the preheated oven for 15-20 minutes, or until mushrooms are tender and cheese is melted.
7. Serve hot, garnished with additional grated Parmesan cheese if desired.

Nutrition Information (per serving):

- Calories: 150

- Protein: 10g

- Carbohydrates: 8g

- Fat: 8g

- Fiber: 2g

- Sugar: 2g

- Portion Size: 1 stuffed portobello mushroom

Baked Cod with Green Beans

Ingredients:

- 4 cod fillets

- 2 cups green beans, trimmed

- 2 tablespoons olive oil

- 2 tablespoons lemon juice

- 2 cloves garlic, minced

- 1 teaspoon dried dill

- Salt and pepper to taste

Instructions:

1. Preheat the oven to 400°F (200°C).

2. Place cod fillets on a baking sheet lined with parchment paper.

3. In a small bowl, whisk together olive oil, lemon juice, minced garlic, dried dill, salt, and pepper.

4. Drizzle the marinade over the cod fillets.

5. Arrange green beans around the cod fillets on the baking sheet.

6. Bake in the preheated oven for 15-20 minutes, or until the cod is cooked through and flakes easily with a fork.

7. Serve hot, with green beans alongside baked cod.

Nutrition Information (per serving):

- Calories: 250
- Protein: 25g
- Carbohydrates: 8g
- Fat: 12g
- Fiber: 3g
- Sugar: 3g
- Portion Size: 1 cod fillet with green beans

Eggplant Parmesan with Whole Wheat Spaghetti

Ingredients:

- 1 large eggplant, sliced into rounds
- 1 cup whole wheat breadcrumbs
- 1/4 cup grated Parmesan cheese
- 2 eggs, beaten
- 2 cups marinara sauce
- 1 cup shredded mozzarella cheese
- Whole wheat spaghetti, cooked according to package instructions
- Fresh basil leaves for garnish

Instructions:

1. Preheat the oven to 375°F (190°C).
2. Dip eggplant slices into beaten eggs, then coat with a mixture of whole wheat breadcrumbs and grated Parmesan cheese.
3. Place coated eggplant slices on a baking sheet lined with parchment paper.

4. Bake in the preheated oven for 20-25 minutes, or until eggplant is tender and breadcrumbs are golden brown.

5. Spread marinara sauce in the bottom of a baking dish.

6. Arrange baked eggplant slices over the marinara sauce.

7. Top each eggplant slice with additional marinara sauce and shredded mozzarella cheese.

8. Bake for an additional 15-20 minutes, or until the cheese is melted and bubbly.

9. Serve hot, with whole wheat spaghetti and garnished with fresh basil leaves.

Nutrition Information (per serving):

- Calories: 380
- Protein: 20g
- Carbohydrates: 45g
- Fat: 15g
- Fiber: 8g
- Sugar: 10g
- Portion Size: 1 cup of eggplant parmesan with spaghetti

Chicken and Vegetable Kebabs with Brown Rice

Ingredients:

- 1 lb boneless, skinless chicken breasts, cut into chunks
- 2 bell peppers, cut into chunks
- 1 red onion, cut into chunks
- 1 zucchini, sliced
- 1/4 cup olive oil
- 2 cloves garlic, minced
- 1 teaspoon dried oregano
- Salt and pepper to taste
- Cooked brown rice for serving

Instructions:

1. In a bowl, combine olive oil, minced garlic, dried oregano, salt, and pepper to make the marinade.
2. Thread chicken, bell peppers, red onion, and zucchini onto skewers.
3. Brush the marinade over the chicken and vegetable skewers.
4. Preheat the grill to medium-high heat.

5. Grill the skewers for 10-12 minutes, turning occasionally, until chicken is cooked through and vegetables are tender.

6. Serve hot, with cooked brown rice.

Nutrition Information (per serving):

- Calories: 320

- Protein: 25g

- Carbohydrates: 20g

- Fat: 15g

- Fiber: 5g

- Sugar: 5g

- Portion Size: 2 skewers with brown rice

Turkey and Vegetable Stir-Fry with Cauliflower Rice

Ingredients:

- 1 lb lean ground turkey

- 2 cups mixed vegetables (such as bell peppers, broccoli, snap peas)

- 1 tablespoon olive oil

- 2 cloves garlic, minced

- 1 tablespoon low-sodium soy sauce

- 1 teaspoon sesame oil

- Salt and pepper to taste

- 4 cups cauliflower rice

Instructions:

1. In a large skillet or wok, heat olive oil over medium-high heat.

2. Add minced garlic to the skillet and cook for 1 minute until fragrant.

3. Add lean ground turkey to the skillet and cook until browned.

4. Add mixed vegetables to the skillet and stir-fry for 3-4 minutes until tender-crisp.

5. Stir in low-sodium soy sauce and sesame oil, and season with salt and pepper to taste.

6. Meanwhile, steam cauliflower rice until tender.

7. Serve turkey and vegetable stir-fry over cauliflower rice.

Nutrition Information (per serving):

- Calories: 280

- Protein: 25g

- Carbohydrates: 15g

- Fat: 12g

- Fiber: 5g

- Sugar: 5g

- Portion Size: 1 cup of turkey and vegetable stir-fry with cauliflower rice

Chapter 5: Snacks and Appetizers

These snacks and appetizers are carefully curated to provide balanced nutrition while satisfying cravings. From crunchy veggies paired with creamy dips to satisfying protein-packed options, these recipes aim to make snacking a guilt-free pleasure for your little ones.

Celery Sticks with Peanut Butter

Ingredients:

- Fresh celery sticks
- Natural peanut butter

Instructions:

1. Wash and cut celery sticks into manageable sizes.
2. Spread peanut butter onto celery sticks.
3. Enjoy!

Nutrition Information:

- Calories: 100
- Protein: 3g

- Carbohydrates: 6g
- Fat: 8g
- Fiber: 3g
- Sugar: 2g
- Portion size: 2 celery sticks with 2 tbsp peanut butter

Guacamole with Carrot Sticks

Ingredients:

- Ripe avocados
- Lime juice
- Diced tomatoes
- Minced garlic
- Chopped cilantro
- Salt and pepper
- Carrot sticks for dipping

Instructions:

1. Mash avocados in a bowl and mix with lime juice.
2. Stir in diced tomatoes, minced garlic, chopped cilantro, salt, and pepper.
3. Serve with carrot sticks for dipping.

Nutrition Information:

- Calories: 120
- Protein: 2g
- Carbohydrates: 8g
- Fat: 10g
- Fiber: 6g
- Sugar: 2g
- Portion size: 1/4 cup guacamole with 1 carrot

Greek Yogurt with Berries

Ingredients:

- Greek yogurt
- Fresh berries (such as strawberries, blueberries, raspberries)

Instructions:

1. Spoon Greek yogurt into a bowl.
2. Top with fresh berries.
3. Enjoy as a creamy and fruity snack!

Nutrition Information:

- Calories: 150

- Protein: 15g
- Carbohydrates: 20g
- Fat: 0g
- Fiber: 3g
- Sugar: 15g
- Portion size: 1/2 cup Greek yogurt with 1/2 cup berries

Cottage Cheese and Pineapple

Ingredients:

- Low-fat cottage cheese
- Fresh pineapple chunks

Instructions:

1. Place cottage cheese in a bowl.
2. Add fresh pineapple chunks on top.
3. Serve chilled for a refreshing snack.

Nutrition Information:

- Calories: 130
- Protein: 14g
- Carbohydrates: 15g

- Fat: 2g
- Fiber: 2g
- Sugar: 12g
- Portion size: 1/2 cup cottage cheese with 1/2 cup pineapple chunks

Hummus and Whole Wheat Pita Chips

Ingredients:

- Hummus (store-bought or homemade)
- Whole wheat pita bread, cut into triangles

Instructions:

1. Spread hummus onto whole wheat pita triangles.
2. Enjoy as a crunchy and satisfying snack!

Nutrition Information:

- Calories: 160
- Protein: 5g
- Carbohydrates: 25g
- Fat: 4g

- Fiber: 6g

- Sugar: 1g

- Portion size: 1/4 cup hummus with 6 whole wheat pita triangles

Trail Mix with Nuts and Seeds

Ingredients:

- Assorted nuts (almonds, cashews, peanuts)

- Assorted seeds (pumpkin seeds, sunflower seeds)

- Dried fruits (raisins, cranberries)

Instructions:

1. Mix together nuts, seeds, and dried fruits in a bowl.

2. Portion into snack-sized bags for convenient munching.

Nutrition Information:

- Calories: 200

- Protein: 7g

- Carbohydrates: 15g

- Fat: 14g

- Fiber: 4g

- Sugar: 8g

- Portion size: 1/4 cup trail mix

Apple Slices with Almond Butter

Ingredients:

- Fresh apple, sliced

- Almond butter

Instructions:

1. Slice apple into wedges.

2. Spread almond butter onto apple slices.

3. Enjoy as a sweet and crunchy snack!

Nutrition Information:

- Calories: 160

- Protein: 3g

- Carbohydrates: 20g

- Fat: 8g

- Fiber: 5g

- Sugar: 14g

- Portion size: 1 medium apple with 2 tbsp almond butter

Edamame with Sea Salt

Ingredients:

- Frozen edamame pods
- Sea salt

Instructions:

1. Boil or steam edamame pods according to package instructions.
2. Sprinkle with sea salt.
3. Enjoy by popping the beans out of the pods.

Nutrition Information:

- Calories: 100
- Protein: 9g
- Carbohydrates: 8g
- Fat: 4g
- Fiber: 4g
- Sugar: 2g
- Portion size: 1/2 cup edamame

Veggie Sticks with Greek Yogurt Dip

Ingredients:

- Assorted vegetable sticks (carrots, cucumber, bell peppers)
- Greek yogurt
- Lemon juice
- Minced garlic
- Dill (fresh or dried)
- Salt and pepper

Instructions:

1. Cut vegetables into sticks.
2. Mix Greek yogurt with lemon juice, minced garlic, dill, salt, and pepper to taste for the dip.
3. Serve the vegetable sticks with the Greek yogurt dip.

Nutrition Information:

- Calories: 70
- Protein: 4g
- Carbohydrates: 10g
- Fat: 1g
- Fiber: 3g

- Sugar: 6g

- Portion size: 1/2 cup vegetable sticks with 1/4 cup Greek yogurt dip

Baked Sweet Potato Fries

Ingredients:

- Sweet potatoes

- Olive oil

- Paprika

- Salt and pepper

Instructions:

1. Preheat oven to 425°F (220°C).

2. Peel and cut sweet potatoes into fries.

3. Toss with olive oil, paprika, salt, and pepper.

4. Arrange in a single layer on a baking sheet.

5. Bake for 25-30 minutes, flipping halfway through, until crispy.

6. Serve hot as a nutritious alternative to regular fries.

Nutrition Information:

- Calories: 120

- Protein: 2g
- Carbohydrates: 25g
- Fat: 2g
- Fiber: 4g
- Sugar: 5g
- Portion size: 1 cup baked sweet potato fries

Cherry Tomatoes with Mozzarella Balls

Ingredients:

- Cherry tomatoes
- Fresh mozzarella balls
- Basil leaves
- Balsamic glaze (optional)

Instructions:

1. Thread cherry tomatoes, mozzarella balls, and basil leaves onto toothpicks or skewers.
2. Drizzle with balsamic glaze if desired.
3. Serve as a colorful and flavorful appetizer.

Nutrition Information:

- Calories: 100
- Protein: 5g
- Carbohydrates: 4g
- Fat: 7g
- Fiber: 1g
- Sugar: 2g
- Portion size: 1 serving (approx. 4 skewers)

Almonds and Dried Fruit

Ingredients:

- Almonds
- Assorted dried fruits (raisins, apricots, cranberries)

Instructions:

1. Mix together almonds and dried fruits in a bowl.
2. Portion into snack-sized bags for easy grab-and-go snacks.

Nutrition Information:

- Calories: 160
- Protein: 5g

- Carbohydrates: 15g

- Fat: 10g

- Fiber: 3g

- Sugar: 10g

- Portion size: 1/4 cup almonds with 1/4 cup dried fruits

Whole Grain Crackers with Cheese

Ingredients:

- Whole grain crackers

- Sliced cheese (such as cheddar, Swiss, or mozzarella)

Instructions:

1. Place sliced cheese on top of whole grain crackers.
2. Enjoy as a satisfying and crunchy snack!

Nutrition Information:

- Calories: 140

- Protein: 6g

- Carbohydrates: 15g

- Fat: 7g

- Fiber: 3g
- Sugar: 1g
- Portion size: 6 whole grain crackers with 1 slice of cheese

Hard-Boiled Eggs

Ingredients:

- Eggs

Instructions:

1. Place eggs in a pot and cover with water.
2. Bring to a boil, then reduce heat and simmer for 10-12 minutes.
3. Remove from heat and place eggs in cold water to cool.
4. Peel and enjoy as a protein-rich snack or appetizer.

Nutrition Information:

- Calories: 70
- Protein: 6g
- Carbohydrates: 1g
- Fat: 5g

- Fiber: 0g

- Sugar: 0g

- Portion size: 1 hard-boiled egg

Cucumber Slices with Tzatziki Sauce

Ingredients:

- Cucumber, thinly sliced

- Greek yogurt

- Grated cucumber

- Minced garlic

- Lemon juice

- Chopped fresh dill

- Salt and pepper

Instructions:

1. Mix Greek yogurt with grated cucumber, minced garlic, lemon juice, chopped dill, salt, and pepper to taste to make tzatziki sauce.

2. Arrange cucumber slices on a plate.

3. Serve with tzatziki sauce for dipping.

Nutrition Information:

- Calories: 60
- Protein: 3g
- Carbohydrates: 8g
- Fat: 2g
- Fiber: 1g
- Sugar: 4g
- Portion size: 1/2 cup cucumber slices with 1/4 cup tzatziki sauce

Chapter 6: Desserts

These desserts are crafted to satisfy sweet cravings while also providing balanced nutrition. From fruity delights to creamy indulgences, each recipe offers a unique combination of flavors and textures that are sure to please young palates.

Berry Yogurt Popsicles

Ingredients:

- 1 cup Greek yogurt
- 1/2 cup mixed berries (such as strawberries, blueberries, raspberries)
- 1 tablespoon honey or maple syrup (optional)

Instructions:

1. In a blender, combine Greek yogurt, mixed berries, and honey or maple syrup.
2. Blend until smooth.
3. Pour the mixture into popsicle molds.

4. Insert popsicle sticks and freeze for at least 4 hours or until solid.

5. Once frozen, remove from molds and enjoy!

Nutrition Information (per serving):

- Calories: 70

- Protein: 5g

- Carbohydrates: 10g

- Fat: 1g

- Fiber: 1g

- Sugar: 8g

- Portion size: 1 popsicle

Dark Chocolate Covered Strawberries

Ingredients:

- 8-10 fresh strawberries

- 1/4 cup dark chocolate chips

- 1 teaspoon coconut oil

Instructions:

1. Wash and dry strawberries, leaving the stems intact.

2. In a microwave-safe bowl, melt dark chocolate chips with coconut oil in 30-second intervals, stirring until smooth.

3. Dip each strawberry into the melted chocolate, coating about halfway.

4. Place dipped strawberries on a parchment-lined baking sheet.

5. Refrigerate for 15-20 minutes or until the chocolate sets.

6. Serve and enjoy!

Nutrition Information (per serving, 2 strawberries):

- Calories: 90
- Protein: 1g
- Carbohydrates: 12g
- Fat: 5g
- Fiber: 2g
- Sugar: 8g
- Portion size: 2 strawberries

Baked Apple Chips

Ingredients:

- 2 large apples, thinly sliced
- 1 tablespoon lemon juice
- 1 teaspoon ground cinnamon

Instructions:

1. Preheat oven to 200°F (95°C).
2. In a bowl, toss apple slices with lemon juice and ground cinnamon until evenly coated.
3. Place apple slices on a parchment-lined baking sheet in a single layer, making sure they do not overlap.
4. Bake for 2-3 hours, flipping halfway through, until apples are dried and crispy.
5. Allow to cool before serving.

Nutrition Information (per serving, 1/2 apple):

- Calories: 50
- Protein: 0g
- Carbohydrates: 14g
- Fat: 0g
- Fiber: 3g

- Sugar: 10g
- Portion size: 1/2 apple

Frozen Banana Bites

Ingredients:

- 2 ripe bananas
- 1/4 cup peanut butter
- 1/4 cup dark chocolate chips

Instructions:

1. Peel bananas and cut them into bite-sized pieces.
2. Spread a thin layer of peanut butter onto half of the banana pieces.
3. Sandwich the remaining banana pieces on top to form banana bites.
4. Place banana bites on a parchment-lined baking sheet and freeze for 1 hour.
5. In a microwave-safe bowl, melt dark chocolate chips in 30-second intervals, stirring until smooth.
6. Dip each frozen banana bite into the melted chocolate, coating halfway.

7. Return to the baking sheet and freeze for an additional 30 minutes or until chocolate sets.

8. Serve cold and enjoy!

Nutrition Information (per serving, 4 banana bites):

- Calories: 140
- Protein: 3g
- Carbohydrates: 20g
- Fat: 7g
- Fiber: 3g
- Sugar: 12g
- Portion size: 4 banana bites

Greek Yogurt Bark with Fruit and Nuts

Ingredients:

- 1 cup plain Greek yogurt
- 2 tablespoons honey or maple syrup
- 1/4 cup mixed fruits (such as strawberries, blueberries, kiwi)

- 2 tablespoons chopped nuts (such as almonds, walnuts)

Instructions:

1. Line a baking sheet with parchment paper.
2. In a bowl, mix Greek yogurt and honey or maple syrup until well combined.
3. Spread the yogurt mixture evenly onto the prepared baking sheet.
4. Sprinkle mixed fruits and chopped nuts over the yogurt.
5. Freeze for 2-3 hours or until firm.
6. Once frozen, break the yogurt bark into pieces and serve immediately.

Nutrition Information (per serving, 1/4 cup):

- Calories: 80
- Protein: 5g
- Carbohydrates: 9g
- Fat: 3g
- Fiber: 1g
- Sugar: 7g

- Portion size: 1/4 cup

Chocolate Avocado Mousse

Ingredients:

- 2 ripe avocados
- 1/4 cup cocoa powder
- 1/4 cup honey or maple syrup
- 1 teaspoon vanilla extract

Instructions:

1. Cut avocados in half, remove pits, and scoop out the flesh into a blender or food processor.
2. Add cocoa powder, honey or maple syrup, and vanilla extract to the blender.
3. Blend until smooth and creamy, scraping down the sides as needed.
4. Transfer the mousse to serving cups or bowls.
5. Refrigerate for at least 1 hour before serving.
6. Garnish with fresh berries or shaved chocolate if desired.
7. Serve chilled and enjoy!

Nutrition Information (per serving, 1/2 cup):

- Calories: 180
- Protein: 3g
- Carbohydrates: 20g
- Fat: 12g
- Fiber: 7g
- Sugar: 10g
- Portion size: 1/2 cup

Rice Cake with Almond Butter and Banana Slices

Ingredients:

- 1 rice cake
- 1 tablespoon almond butter
- 1/2 ripe banana, sliced

Instructions:

1. Spread almond butter evenly onto the rice cake.
2. Arrange banana slices on top of the almond butter.
3. Serve immediately and enjoy!

Nutrition Information (per serving, 1 rice cake):

- Calories: 120
- Protein: 3g
- Carbohydrates: 18g
- Fat: 5g
- Fiber: 2g
- Sugar: 7g
- Portion size: 1 rice cake

Baked Pear with Cinnamon

Ingredients:

- 1 ripe pear
- 1/2 teaspoon ground cinnamon

Instructions:

1. Preheat oven to 350°F (175°C).
2. Cut pear in half and remove the core.
3. Place pear halves on a baking sheet, cut side up.
4. Sprinkle ground cinnamon evenly over the pear halves.
5. Bake for 20-25 minutes or until pear is tender.
6. Serve warm and enjoy!

Nutrition Information (per serving, 1 pear half):

- Calories: 60
- Protein: 0g
- Carbohydrates: 16g
- Fat: 0g
- Fiber: 3g
- Sugar: 9g
- Portion size: 1 pear half

Oatmeal Raisin Cookies with Whole Grains

Ingredients:

- 1 cup old-fashioned oats
- 1/2 cup whole wheat flour
- 1/4 teaspoon baking soda
- 1/4 teaspoon ground cinnamon
- 1/4 cup unsweetened applesauce
- 1/4 cup honey or maple syrup
- 1/4 cup raisins

Instructions:

1. Preheat oven to 350°F (175°C) and line a baking sheet with parchment paper.
2. In a mixing bowl, combine oats, whole wheat flour, baking soda, and ground cinnamon.
3. Add unsweetened applesauce and honey or maple syrup to the dry ingredients, mixing until well combined.
4. Fold in raisins.
5. Drop spoonfuls of the cookie dough onto the prepared baking sheet, spacing them apart.
6. Flatten each cookie slightly with the back of a spoon.
7. Bake for 10-12 minutes or until golden brown.
8. Allow cookies to cool on the baking sheet for 5 minutes before transferring to a wire rack to cool completely.

Nutrition Information (per serving, 1 cookie):

- Calories: 70
- Protein: 1g
- Carbohydrates: 15g
- Fat: 1g

- Fiber: 1g

- Sugar: 6g

- Portion size: 1 cookie

Pumpkin Pie Smoothie

Ingredients:

- 1/2 cup canned pumpkin puree

- 1/2 cup plain Greek yogurt

- 1/2 cup unsweetened almond milk

- 1/2 teaspoon ground cinnamon

- 1/4 teaspoon ground nutmeg

- 1 tablespoon honey or maple syrup (optional)

- 1/2 cup ice cubes

Instructions:

1. In a blender, combine canned pumpkin puree, Greek yogurt, almond milk, ground cinnamon, ground nutmeg, and honey or maple syrup.

2. Add ice cubes to the blender.

3. Blend until smooth and creamy.

4. Pour into glasses and serve immediately.

Nutrition Information (per serving):

- Calories: 80
- Protein: 5g
- Carbohydrates: 13g
- Fat: 2g
- Fiber: 3g
- Sugar: 7g
- Portion size: 1 cup

Coconut Chia Seed Pudding

Ingredients:

- 1/4 cup chia seeds
- 1 cup coconut milk
- 1 tablespoon honey or maple syrup
- 1/4 teaspoon vanilla extract
- Unsweetened shredded coconut, for garnish (optional)
- Fresh berries, for garnish (optional)

Instructions:

1. In a bowl, mix chia seeds, coconut milk, honey or maple syrup, and vanilla extract.

2. Stir well to combine.

3. Cover the bowl and refrigerate for at least 2 hours or overnight, until the mixture thickens and becomes pudding-like.

4. Stir the pudding before serving.

5. Garnish with unsweetened shredded coconut and fresh berries, if desired.

6. Serve chilled and enjoy!

Nutrition Information (per serving):

- Calories: 160
- Protein: 3g
- Carbohydrates: 13g
- Fat: 11g
- Fiber: 8g
- Sugar: 4g
- Portion size: 1/2 cup

Peach and Berry Cobbler with Oat Topping

Ingredients:

- 2 cups sliced peaches (fresh or frozen)
- 1 cup mixed berries (such as strawberries, blueberries, raspberries)
- 1 tablespoon honey or maple syrup
- 1/2 teaspoon ground cinnamon
- 1/2 cup old-fashioned oats
- 1/4 cup whole wheat flour
- 2 tablespoons unsalted butter, melted
- 2 tablespoons honey or maple syrup

Instructions:

1. Preheat oven to 350°F (175°C).
2. In a mixing bowl, combine sliced peaches, mixed berries, honey or maple syrup, and ground cinnamon.
3. Transfer the fruit mixture to a baking dish.
4. In a separate bowl, mix oats, whole wheat flour, melted butter, and honey or maple syrup until crumbly.

5. Sprinkle the oat topping evenly over the fruit mixture.

6. Bake for 30-35 minutes or until the topping is golden brown and the fruit is bubbling.

7. Allow to cool slightly before serving.

8. Serve warm and enjoy!

Nutrition Information (per serving):

- Calories: 150

- Protein: 2g

- Carbohydrates: 28g

- Fat: 5g

- Fiber: 4g

- Sugar: 17g

- Portion size: 1/2 cup

Mango Sorbet with Fresh Mint

Ingredients:

- 2 cups frozen mango chunks

- 1/4 cup fresh mint leaves

- 1-2 tablespoons honey or maple syrup (optional)

- 1/4 cup water

Instructions:

1. In a blender or food processor, combine frozen mango chunks, fresh mint leaves, honey or maple syrup (if using), and water.

2. Blend until smooth and creamy, adding more water if needed to reach desired consistency.

3. Transfer the mixture to a shallow dish and spread it evenly.

4. Cover and freeze for at least 2 hours or until firm.

5. Once frozen, scoop the sorbet into bowls and garnish with fresh mint leaves.

6. Serve immediately and enjoy!

Nutrition Information (per serving):

- Calories: 90
- Protein: 1g
- Carbohydrates: 23g
- Fat: 0g
- Fiber: 3g
- Sugar: 20g
- Portion size: 1/2 cup

Strawberry Banana Frozen Yogurt

Ingredients:

- 2 cups frozen strawberries
- 1 ripe banana
- 1/2 cup plain Greek yogurt
- 1-2 tablespoons honey or maple syrup (optional)
- 1/4 teaspoon vanilla extract

Instructions:

1. In a blender or food processor, combine frozen strawberries, ripe banana, Greek yogurt, honey or maple syrup (if using), and vanilla extract.
2. Blend until smooth and creamy, scraping down the sides as needed.
3. Transfer the mixture to a shallow dish and spread it evenly.
4. Cover and freeze for at least 2 hours or until firm.
5. Once frozen, scoop the frozen yogurt into bowls and serve immediately.

Nutrition Information (per serving):

- Calories: 100

- Protein: 3g
- Carbohydrates: 22g
- Fat: 0g
- Fiber: 3g
- Sugar: 16g
- Portion size: 1/2 cup

Carrot Cake Energy Bites

Ingredients:

- 1 cup rolled oats
- 1/2 cup shredded carrots
- 1/4 cup almond butter
- 1/4 cup honey or maple syrup
- 1/4 cup chopped walnuts
- 1/4 cup raisins
- 1/2 teaspoon ground cinnamon
- 1/4 teaspoon ground nutmeg
- 1/4 teaspoon vanilla extract
- Pinch of salt

Instructions:

1. In a mixing bowl, combine rolled oats, shredded carrots, almond butter, honey or maple syrup, chopped walnuts, raisins, ground cinnamon, ground nutmeg, vanilla extract, and a pinch of salt.
2. Mix until well combined and the mixture holds together.
3. Roll the mixture into bite-sized balls using your hands.
4. Place the energy bites on a parchment-lined baking sheet.
5. Refrigerate for at least 30 minutes to firm up.
6. Once firm, transfer the energy bites to an airtight container and store in the refrigerator.
7. Enjoy as a healthy and energy-boosting snack!

Nutrition Information (per serving, 1 energy bite):

- Calories: 80
- Protein: 2g
- Carbohydrates: 10g
- Fat: 4g
- Fiber: 1g

- Sugar: 5g
- Portion size: 1 energy bite

Chapter 7: Smoothies

Smoothies are not only a convenient way to incorporate essential nutrients into your child's diet but also offer a refreshing and satisfying treat. Packed with vitamins, minerals, and fiber, these smoothies provide a wholesome option for breakfast, snack time, or any time of the day.

Green Smoothie with Spinach and Pineapple

Ingredients:

- 1 cup fresh spinach leaves
- 1 cup diced pineapple
- 1 banana, peeled
- 1/2 cup unsweetened almond milk
- Ice cubes (optional)

Instructions:

1. Place spinach, pineapple, banana, and almond milk in a blender.
2. Blend until smooth and creamy.

3. Add ice cubes if desired and blend again until well combined.

4. Pour into glasses and serve immediately.

Nutrition Information (per serving):

- Calories: 120

- Protein: 3g

- Carbohydrates: 28g

- Fat: 1g

- Fiber: 4g

- Sugar: 18g

- Portion size: 1 cup

Berry Blast Smoothie with Greek Yogurt

Ingredients:

- 1 cup mixed berries (such as strawberries, blueberries, raspberries)

- 1/2 cup plain Greek yogurt

- 1/2 cup unsweetened almond milk

- 1 tablespoon honey (optional)

- Ice cubes (optional)

Instructions:

1. Combine mixed berries, Greek yogurt, almond milk, and honey (if using) in a blender.
2. Blend until smooth and creamy.
3. Add ice cubes if desired and blend again until well mixed.
4. Pour into glasses and serve immediately.

Nutrition Information (per serving):

- Calories: 150
- Protein: 8g
- Carbohydrates: 25g
- Fat: 3g
- Fiber: 5g
- Sugar: 18g
- Portion size: 1 cup

Tropical Paradise Smoothie with Mango and Coconut

Ingredients:

- 1 cup diced mango
- 1/2 cup coconut milk
- 1/2 cup unsweetened pineapple juice
- 1 banana, peeled
- Ice cubes (optional)

Instructions:

1. Place diced mango, coconut milk, pineapple juice, and banana in a blender.
2. Blend until smooth and creamy.
3. Add ice cubes if desired and blend again until well incorporated.
4. Pour into glasses and serve immediately.

Nutrition Information (per serving):

- Calories: 180
- Protein: 2g
- Carbohydrates: 35g
- Fat: 5g

- Fiber: 3g
- Sugar: 25g
- Portion size: 1 cup

Chocolate Banana Smoothie with Almond Milk

Ingredients:

- 1 ripe banana
- 1 tablespoon unsweetened cocoa powder
- 1 cup unsweetened almond milk
- 1/2 teaspoon vanilla extract
- Ice cubes (optional)

Instructions:

1. Peel the banana and place it in a blender.
2. Add cocoa powder, almond milk, and vanilla extract.
3. Blend until smooth and creamy.
4. If desired, add ice cubes and blend again until well combined.
5. Pour into glasses and serve immediately.

Nutrition Information (per serving):

- Calories: 130
- Protein: 2g
- Carbohydrates: 25g
- Fat: 3g
- Fiber: 5g
- Sugar: 12g
- Portion size: 1 cup

Peanut Butter and Banana Smoothie

Ingredients:

- 1 ripe banana
- 2 tablespoons natural peanut butter
- 1 cup unsweetened almond milk
- 1 tablespoon honey (optional)
- Ice cubes (optional)

Instructions:

1. Peel the banana and place it in a blender.
2. Add peanut butter, almond milk, and honey (if using).
3. Blend until smooth and creamy.

4. Add ice cubes if desired and blend again until well mixed.

5. Pour into glasses and serve immediately.

Nutrition Information (per serving):

- Calories: 250

- Protein: 7g

- Carbohydrates: 20g

- Fat: 15g

- Fiber: 3g

- Sugar: 10g

- Portion size: 1 cup

Kale and Kiwi Smoothie with Orange Juice

Ingredients:

- 1 cup chopped kale leaves

- 2 kiwis, peeled and diced

- 1/2 cup orange juice

- 1/2 cup plain Greek yogurt

- Ice cubes (optional)

Instructions:

1. Place kale, kiwi, orange juice, and Greek yogurt in a blender.
2. Blend until smooth and creamy.
3. If desired, add ice cubes and blend again until well incorporated.
4. Pour into glasses and serve immediately.

Nutrition Information (per serving):

- Calories: 140
- Protein: 7g
- Carbohydrates: 30g
- Fat: 1g
- Fiber: 5g
- Sugar: 18g
- Portion size: 1 cup

Blueberry Almond Smoothie with Flaxseed

Ingredients:

- 1 cup frozen blueberries

- 1/4 cup almonds
- 1 tablespoon ground flaxseed
- 1/2 cup unsweetened almond milk
- Ice cubes (optional)

Instructions:

1. Combine frozen blueberries, almonds, flaxseed, and almond milk in a blender.
2. Blend until smooth and creamy.
3. Add ice cubes if desired and blend again until well mixed.
4. Pour into glasses and serve immediately.

Nutrition Information (per serving):

- Calories: 180
- Protein: 6g
- Carbohydrates: 20g
- Fat: 10g
- Fiber: 6g
- Sugar: 10g
- Portion size: 1 cup

Pineapple Mango Smoothie with Spinach

Ingredients:

- 1 cup diced pineapple
- 1 cup diced mango
- Handful of fresh spinach leaves
- 1/2 cup coconut water
- Ice cubes (optional)

Instructions:

1. Place diced pineapple, mango, spinach, and coconut water in a blender.
2. Blend until smooth and creamy.
3. Add ice cubes if desired and blend again until well incorporated.
4. Pour into glasses and serve immediately.

Nutrition Information (per serving):

- Calories: 160
- Protein: 3g
- Carbohydrates: 35g
- Fat: 1g

- Fiber: 5g

- Sugar: 25g

- Portion size: 1 cup

Avocado Spinach Smoothie with Honey

Ingredients:

- 1/2 ripe avocado

- Handful of fresh spinach leaves

- 1/2 cup plain Greek yogurt

- 1 tablespoon honey

- 1/2 cup unsweetened almond milk

- Ice cubes (optional)

Instructions:

1. Scoop out the avocado flesh and place it in a blender.

2. Add spinach, Greek yogurt, honey, and almond milk.

3. Blend until smooth and creamy.

4. If desired, add ice cubes and blend again until well mixed.

5. Pour into glasses and serve immediately.

Nutrition Information (per serving):

- Calories: 200
- Protein: 8g
- Carbohydrates: 20g
- Fat: 10g
- Fiber: 5g
- Sugar: 10g
- Portion size: 1 cup

Raspberry Peach Smoothie with Greek Yogurt

Ingredients:

- 1 cup frozen raspberries
- 1 ripe peach, pitted and diced
- 1/2 cup plain Greek yogurt
- 1/2 cup unsweetened almond milk
- Ice cubes (optional)

Instructions:

1. Combine frozen raspberries, diced peach, Greek yogurt, and almond milk in a blender.

2. Blend until smooth and creamy.

3. Add ice cubes if desired and blend again until well mixed.

4. Pour into glasses and serve immediately.

Nutrition Information (per serving):

- Calories: 150

- Protein: 8g

- Carbohydrates: 25g

- Fat: 3g

- Fiber: 8g

- Sugar: 15g

- Portion size: 1 cup

Beetroot and Berry Smoothie

Ingredients:

- 1 small beetroot, peeled and diced

- 1/2 cup mixed berries (such as strawberries, blueberries, raspberries)

- 1/2 cup plain Greek yogurt

- 1/2 cup unsweetened almond milk

- 1 tablespoon honey (optional)

- Ice cubes (optional)

Instructions:

1. Place diced beetroot, mixed berries, Greek yogurt, almond milk, and honey (if using) in a blender.
2. Blend until smooth and creamy.
3. If desired, add ice cubes and blend again until well incorporated.
4. Pour into glasses and serve immediately.

Nutrition Information (per serving):

- Calories: 170
- Protein: 9g
- Carbohydrates: 30g
- Fat: 2g
- Fiber: 6g
- Sugar: 20g
- Portion size: 1 cup

Carrot Orange Smoothie with Ginger

Ingredients:

- 1 large carrot, peeled and chopped

- Juice of 2 oranges
- 1/2 inch fresh ginger, peeled and grated
- 1/2 cup plain Greek yogurt
- 1/2 cup unsweetened almond milk
- Ice cubes (optional)

Instructions:

1. Combine chopped carrot, orange juice, grated ginger, Greek yogurt, and almond milk in a blender.
2. Blend until smooth and creamy.
3. Add ice cubes if desired and blend again until well mixed.
4. Pour into glasses and serve immediately.

Nutrition Information (per serving):

- Calories: 140
- Protein: 7g
- Carbohydrates: 25g
- Fat: 2g
- Fiber: 4g
- Sugar: 18g
- Portion size: 1 cup

Cucumber Mint Smoothie with Lime

Ingredients:

- 1 cucumber, peeled and diced
- Handful of fresh mint leaves
- Juice of 1 lime
- 1/2 cup plain Greek yogurt
- 1/2 cup coconut water
- Ice cubes (optional)

Instructions:

1. Place diced cucumber, mint leaves, lime juice, Greek yogurt, and coconut water in a blender.
2. Blend until smooth and creamy.
3. If desired, add ice cubes and blend again until well incorporated.
4. Pour into glasses and serve immediately.

Nutrition Information (per serving):

- Calories: 120
- Protein: 7g
- Carbohydrates: 20g
- Fat: 1g

- Fiber: 3g
- Sugar: 10g
- Portion size: 1 cup

Cherry Vanilla Smoothie with Almond Milk

Ingredients:

- 1 cup frozen cherries
- 1/2 teaspoon vanilla extract
- 1 cup unsweetened almond milk
- 1/2 cup plain Greek yogurt
- 1 tablespoon honey (optional)
- Ice cubes (optional)

Instructions:

1. Combine frozen cherries, vanilla extract, almond milk, Greek yogurt, and honey (if using) in a blender.
2. Blend until smooth and creamy.
3. Add ice cubes if desired and blend again until well mixed.
4. Pour into glasses and serve immediately.

Nutrition Information (per serving):

- Calories: 160
- Protein: 7g
- Carbohydrates: 25g
- Fat: 3g
- Fiber: 5g
- Sugar: 15g
- Portion size: 1 cup

Protein Power Smoothie with Peanut Butter and Oats

Ingredients:

- 1 banana, peeled
- 2 tablespoons natural peanut butter
- 1/4 cup rolled oats
- 1 cup unsweetened almond milk
- Ice cubes (optional)

Instructions:

1. Peel the banana and place it in a blender.
2. Add peanut butter, rolled oats, and almond milk.

3. Blend until smooth and creamy.

4. If desired, add ice cubes and blend again until well combined.

5. Pour into glasses and serve immediately.

Nutrition Information (per serving):

- Calories: 280

- Protein: 10g

- Carbohydrates: 30g

- Fat: 14g

- Fiber: 6g

- Sugar: 15g

- Portion size: 1 cup

CONCLUSION

"Type 2 Diabetes Cookbook for Kids" serves as a vital resource for families navigating the challenges of managing diabetes in children while ensuring they enjoy delicious, nutritious meals. Through careful planning and creativity, this cookbook offers a diverse array of recipes spanning breakfast, lunch, dinner, snacks, desserts, and smoothies, all tailored to stabilize blood sugar levels and promote overall health.

By emphasizing whole, nutrient-rich ingredients and mindful portion control, this cookbook empowers parents and caregivers to provide balanced meals that not only meet the dietary needs of children with type 2 diabetes but also delight their taste buds. From hearty breakfasts to satisfying dinners, and from wholesome snacks to indulgent desserts, each recipe is thoughtfully crafted to strike the perfect balance between flavor and healthfulness.

Moreover, the inclusion of a 30-day meal plan provides a roadmap for establishing sustainable eating habits, ensuring that families can navigate their diabetes management journey with confidence and ease. With an emphasis on variety, convenience, and culinary creativity, this cookbook encourages experimentation in the kitchen while instilling a lifelong appreciation for wholesome eating habits.

Ultimately, "Type 2 Diabetes Cookbook for Kids" is more than just a collection of recipes; it's a comprehensive guide that empowers families to take control of their health and well-being. By fostering a positive relationship with food and instilling healthy eating habits from an early age, this cookbook paves the way for a lifetime of good health and vitality for children living with type 2 diabetes.